KILLING THE CANCER BEAST

"The Real story of A Woman who was left with
no hope after she was diagnosed with Cancer.
An actual fight of her and her family with the only
weapons which were left to them: love,
strong will and a belief that God should have
thought of an antidote before humans would"

First printing April 2009

ISBN: 978-960-931247-9

DISCLAIMER: While all care is taken with the accuracy of the facts and procedures in this book, the author accept neither liability nor resposibility to any person with respect to loss, injury or damage caused, or alleged to be caused directly or indirectly, by the information contained in this book. The purpose of this book is to educate and inform. For medical advice you should seek the individual, personal advice and services of a health care professional.

Maria D. Georga

KILLING THE CANCER BEAST

A real story

Effective Natural & Mental Tools vs. Cancer

ATHENS 2009

*"Dedicated to the ones who fought cancer and won.
Dedicated to the ones who had the courage to fight
bravely but lost the battle.
Dedicated to the ones who dedicated their lives in research in
order to save human beings from cancer suffering"*

CONTENTS

ACKNOWLEDGMENTS

I am indebted to the many researchers & scientists who have made so much dedicated work on research for foods curing from cancer. These include Dr. Linus Pauling, Dr Levine, and Dr. G. Edward Griffin, Dr. Ernst Krebs and Dr. Batmanghelidg. Also Dr Ihaleakala S. Hew Len for his work on the power of memories.

INTRODUCTION

What I remember from these days are so badly engraved in my mind, I remember everything but most of the times I see myself like somebody else, as if I was not really there, as if somebody else experienced these days just like the human mind reacts after days of hard crises. We feel like needing to escape from negative memories, negative past.

And some times we realize the Murphy's Law is a reality and all sad stories happen the same time period one after the other and this makes us worry: Doesn't life have black humor?

And there I was. A very stressed time of my life with a lot of uncertainties about my life, an extremely highly demanding job with various problems were everybody seemed to count on me and expect from me and yes, this happened.

CHAPTER ONE

My mother Angela, all her life so far used to be one of the healthiest people I knew. I hardly remember her with flu or anything. On the contrary, she was the strong, caring presence taking care of everybody else in the house, me, my two older sisters, my brother and our father when we were ill or happen to break any of our bones while playing during our childhood and later during sports and other accidents. Even with our old grandparents, who by the way all of them had a long living, my mother had invented recipes to keep them healthy and strong and always could find a way to help them deal with their illnesses. Therefore they all gave her their special blessings before they passed away which I believe contributed later in combination with the efforts which we the alive part of the family made in order to help her recover from cancer and keep her with us.

She was fifty-five years old when it all started. A cyst appeared on her right breast. Her healthy appearance, the absence of pain and the lack of cancer history in her family confused her doctors and due to that they kept on emptying the cyst again and again and kept examining the findings that led to an important lose of time. After the last biopsy the doctor just gave her the papers and rather frustrated indicated her to go and stop worrying because "nothing was wrong with her". It was me who took her to other specialized doctors and they all confirmed that she should have surgery in order to get some clean results of the cause of the cyst. Due to our initiative the surgeon lazily gave us a date for the surgery while reassuring us that there is nothing to worry about.

I remember staying calm and the day of the surgery I also went to my office believing that there was nothing to worry about. But it seems that there is indeed a strong bond that develops among family members and between people who have really loved each other that notifies people about everything without words and telephones. My eyes started crying, worries and fear crossed my heart, my mood changed to sadness. I knew I had to be there. When I arrived at the hospital my family was out of the surgery room and three hours had pass already. My father still believed that things where okay since the doctor had agreed to update him during the surgery if something was wrong. But, he did not.

A few minutes after I arrived, the doors opened and the doctors called us in. *"Big cancer tumor hidden, we could not see before", "breast removal", "could not do different", "useless to update you before", "we had to proceed",* were some of the sentences I still remember them saying. I kept on being calm and asked for how long could it be there growing, but no satisfying answer was given to me.

We were all so unprepared. Nobody had given us the real options. It could be a good but it could be a bad tumor. The real options were now coming like a fast down-loading in my mind, one after the other. I had somebody suffering from cancer in my family, my mother, would she make it, would she not, how would my life be after that, what about my father, how could he possibly deal with it, what about her, how are we going to tell her, how is she going to feel, how are we going to help her, if she will not make it how is the family going to cope with it, God she is still so young!

I am ashamed to say it, but I went to her room after one hour. It was impossible for me to see her and not to cry and even more to tell her what had happened. My sister did that tough work.

Surprisingly my mother did not cry, she didn't even look sad and she just said: "All the times, we say it happened to somebody else, this time it happened to me" and then words of pessimism: "We lived our lives, we brought up four children in this world, we did our social duties for our old parents".

There is real tragedy in life sometimes, two days be-fore her surgery her father had passed away. She used to be his favorite daughter and until his last moments he was happy to have her by his side. Through her words it was as if she was saying that it was time for her to go but I didn't let her finish. The encouraging work had just started. The work through which you transfuse a part of your courage, the biggest one, a part of your strength, to someone else who you love and really want to keep at any cost.

The following days I remember myself becoming like made from steel. All emotions were restricted. Getting myself out of bed in the morning, going to work, facing and controlling hard business situations, running to the hospital with my sweetest, childish, optimistic smile, going back to the house late in the night to prepare and have a home dinner with my father, speak with him, encourage him, plant some faith in him. The illness of my mother gave me the ability to discover another side of my father's personality. In my whole life so far I never expected to see that huge man, huge in and out, to collapse, I would never forget the sadness on his face, the pain. With my mother they used to be a couple of beautiful people, married very young and evolved themselves together. Of course they had different personalities. His rather Buddhist, calm, stress less view of life was always contradicted with her social and *"comme il faut"*, stressful view of life, therefore they never missed these repeating arguments mainly about the same reasons. At the bottom line I think that these contradictions were the main challenge to keep this relationship going all their lives. It always surprised me every time they were coming back from an event he would always say: "my lady was nicer than everybody else". My mother was never offered so generous and flattering compliments but from her statements from time to time she seemed to know that her husband was a snip. Ever since all of us left our house I think that my parents redefined their relationship and they came closer to one another as it happens with all couples that have shared important things together during their lives.

Ancient Greeks were saying that there is no Harm that is not followed by Good. An illness in the family is one of the most effective ways to affirm the authenticity of love and friendship of other people toward the person that is suffering and the family. For me it was one of the most accurate, quick and infallible tests. I remember that there were close friends and especially relatives, which in the past enjoyed great support by my family and never show up to a visit at the hospital but at the same time there were people who hardly knew us which called or visited my mother for encouraging her.

This uneasy era did not finish there for me. What our parents taught us about help and altruistic support to weak people and people suffering, in practice didn't work for me. At my work some of my worst competitors thought that it would be a great opportunity for them to attack me in any legit or unethical way. Of course this was the only chance they would ever have to harm me and they knew it. It seemed that I had no other option. I had to fight with everything all together up to the end.

As for my mother, the poor woman lost her breast but the biopsies indicated that although the diseased area was just beside the breast area, this was not an ordinary type of breast cancer. It was a type of cancer rarely met, very aggressive, already found in the worst stage. We were also informed that she had negative adaptors to medicine and therapies and due to the x-rays the oncologist informed me that a new tumor seemed to be created on her shoulder. There was no hope coming from anywhere and nobody seemed willing to help. Then I realized that I had two options: either to leave things in the fatalistic way that most of patients and doctors did in the chemotherapy sections of the hospitals, or to take things in my hands. I think that the second option was more familiar to me.

CHAPTER TWO

Soon after that, I left my job. My loyal companion and I devoted ourselves to finding alternative cancer therapies throughout the globe. I do not even remember how many books we read, how many emails we exchanged with people cured from cancer or alternative therapists, how many hours we devoted on that research and how much money we really spent.

It was a time consuming effort, with no guarantees for the results and only few things kept me going. The love for my mother, my life aspect that there are no limits to anything, and this weird stubborn character that God gave to me when he decided to send me around.

Yes my mother was saved. Despite the pessimistic predictions and the scientific explanations. The doctors out of surprise kept on asking her if she was taking any injection that made her blood so good, indicative of a healthy person. This was the same surprise I faced after the first full tests when my mother proved to be CANCER FREE. It was happiness and satisfaction.

The reason that I proceeded with writing and publishing this book is complex. Since a member of my family was diagnosed and suffered from cancer I am aware of all the feelings that a family and a diseased person faces including physical and emotional extensions.

Also, since God rewarded me with the result of all that hard work by saving my mother, I feel deeply a strong obligation to share with other people my experience and my findings.

This book does not aim to substitute the methods of modern medical science but provides readers some alternatives which can be followed simultaneously with their therapy or as a last chance therapy when medical science therapies are not applicable anymore or do not result to healing a person suffering from cancer. It also aims to give hope to the ones that need it.

In the following pages I will present you one by one all natural products involved in my mother's therapy followed with their special characteristics and a complete explanation of how they affect the body and fight cancer. Also, I will try to point out the importance of good psychology and real encouragement for people suffering.

Studying most therapeutic theories all over the world and starting from ancient Greece with popular Asclepios the first and most popular therapist of the ancient world which use to heal people with herbs I found out that in the nature there are antidotes and cures for every disease.

My interest was fist captured by vitamin C[1]. A vitamin contained in a lot of fruits, vegetables and seeds. I was surprised to read the story of Dr. Linus Pauling, the two-time Nobel laureate who cured himself with intravenous doses of this vitamin. He was diagnosed with cancer and at the last stage. Doctors did not give him even the foggiest hope that he would live. He indeed died but long - long time after that, when he was very old and it was his time to go. Dr. Pauling's life experience encouraged me to keep on with an in depth research of information and definitely for proof. I came in touch with a lot of people who also cured themselves or their beloved with vitamin C over dose. It was not that I had nothing to lose anymore. I was convinced that I only had something to gain. As soon as I found the appropriate type of crystal vitamin C it became a part of my mother's regimen. **Desperate, ill people are open to hope like a mouth waiting for a kiss.** In old times my mother used to be very critical with medicines and vitamins but now she had become an easy going, compliant collaborate to my vision and efforts to keep her with us.

Going deeper with that research the following months, I was amazed from the incredible wealth of cures that exist in the nature. What magnificence! I studied about the miraculous way that enzymes work within the human body, about the selective toxicity of apricot kernels[2] and how cancer cells are specifically targeted and destroyed by the use of vitamin B17. How cyanide who is mainly renown as toxic is targeting the cancer cells and only. For those of you who will obtain this book seeking for detailed knowledge and explanations about the use of natural resources against cancer, you will find an especially analytic, accurate and scientific selection of all official resources on which I based my mother's regimen, on the last Appendixes Chapter of this book. It would be unfair for all these scientists who spent years of their life on scientific search, sometimes on eras where their work was not really being appreciated or faced various difficulties, not to be extensively mentioned and honored by this book. One of these people is Dr. Krebs a chemist who after a long search dared to write a book "World without cancer" who had been stamped as a failure in the time of 70's but not anymore.

I also was deeply impressed by the longevity of Hunza, a tiny kingdom in the remote recesses of the Himalayan Mountains, between West Pakistan, India and China. They live well beyond 100 years and have commonly been known to still father children at the age of 110. The outcome of a big study over this tribe was:

"The Hunza has no known incidence of cancer. They have an abundant crop of apricots. These they dry in the sun and use largely in their food". And "It is important to know when the Hunza leave their secluded land and adopt the menus of other countries, they soon succumb to the same diseases and infirmities including cancer as the rest of man kind."

I also was excited of how these people appreciated the use of apricots in everything like cuisine, cosmetics and medicine. In financial terms, a Hunza man's wealth is defined by the amount of apricot trees he owns and they use to consume apricots and all its products like kernels and apricot oil.

I had become a really passionate student of apricot natural chemistry and its actions in healthy living and especially in cancer fighting. As soon as I found these kernels they also became a part of my mother's everyday diet. Initially started with a few kernels per day and later since she was not affected by any kind of toxicity she almost reached the amount of seeds contained in a daily Hunza's diet. Out of curiosity and driven by a slight fear of cancer heredity I also take them myself from time to time mixed in a jar with honey.

I also came across other nations and tribes who involved a lot of vitamin B17 in their diet like Eskimos, Hopi and Navajo Indians and Abkhazians and they all seemed to have the lowest to zero statistics in cancer. The reason that led me to apricot kernels is that they are the richest food in this very special vitamin.

A dark colored extract mainly coming from Russia soon became a part of my mother's natural regimen. Mumijo Deputatus usually met as Mumio.

The usual conspiracy of the universe made it happen and I found myself in a rather international dinner party with people from allover the world and from the Russia as well. There I heard for first time about this unique extract, which helps almost to every disease from gastric ulcer to cancer. I studied a lot of searches about this black natural extract with the rather weird taste. One of the most valuable effects over the human body is that this extract strengthens the immune system and maintains the blood composition in the appropriate condition as it is in healthy, cancer free people. Especially for people who are under chemotherapy, Mumio is valuable since it provides a strong immune system able to take on the negative effects of chemotherapy, which cannot target on cancer cells only but also destroys healthy cells. Therefore a lot of patients who are under chemo very often have to postpone their scheduled appointment due to the weak condition of their blood, as shown in their blood tests taken prior to a chemo. Mumio is also among the best regimens for a quicker healing of broken bones, arteries and vain cleaning, internal burns and others. I also used it myself during these difficult times when I had to act like a superwoman and deal with all these demands of my life. I was indeed looking and feeling healthy all the way. As for my mother she kept on saying how healthy, fresh and not ill or exhausted she was really feeling and this is what other people who were visiting us could see as well. Mumio is a great confirmation that God has hidden all antidotes in nature and what we have to do is discover them.

During this period and later, a true story that my grandparents use to tell us crossed my mind many times. An old woman, who lived in their village, use to cure everybody with herbs, kernels, droppings from birds and even living bloodsuckers. Once, she cured her worst enemy who use to call her a witch. His face was swollen terribly. Modern medicines and doctors of that era could not do anything but he still refused to let her visit him. At the end when he was left hopeless and desperate and although he was ashamed, he called her as his last chance. She went to him, examined his face carefully with the eyes carrying the wisdom of centuries, the humbleness of a simple woman of the village and the generosity of somebody who is aware that everything belongs to the universe and not to us, and then said: "it seems to be too late but with the help of God I will try". She ran back to her house and came back with a jar of living bloodsuckers. She put a few of them under his eyes along the swollen areas, repeating for a few days. The bloodsuckers started absorbing all dead blood and trapped liquids from this area. His relatives were surprised to see his face entirely restoring and the man got up off his bed. She also gave him a hand made fabric tick containing a coin and recommended him to tie it under his eye, just like a pirate for a few weeks in order for his eye to restore its shape because it looked kind of fallen. My grandfather told me that this man did not follow this last instruction and therefore for the rest of his life one of his eyes seemed to be in a lower position than the other one.

There were also two other experiences of my grandmother with that "therapist" who cured her when some kind of weird, painful, big pimples appeared over her body. The first time she recommended to put some chicken droppings on the pimple. My grandmother who was just a young girl at that time did not want to do it but her mother forced her to. A few hours later, the same afternoon, this pimple swelled up and broke and nothing was left in it. Next morning my grandmother woke up with not even a mark on her skin. She was entirely cured. The second time that something like this happened to her, her mother took her to the house of the old lady. She looked my grandmother's skin. Then she opened a jar containing almonds and gave her a handful of them. Although my grandmother was pleased that she would eat the almonds that she liked so much, the woman told her "chew only and don't swallow". To the disappointment of my grandmother she didn't eat any of the almonds but was asked to put the "chewed paste" on the affected area. But yes she was cured again. That simple.

I cannot retrieve other stories I was told during my childhood and later but I clearly remember that this woman was uneducated and nobody around knew where her knowledge came from. All the people remember seeing her in the fields, on the hills and mountains and aside the creeks most eras of the year collecting her special "medicines". Later on when I happened to deal among others with metempsychosis theory I was convinced that this woman was probably the metempsychosis of an old Indian doctor or even the Greek Asclepios.

Dr. F. Batmanghelidj also impressed me with his theory of cancer cause and natural cure. Through his books[3] I was given an amazing explanation of how valuable water is for someone's body and how dehydration acts against our body in many ways. I also got plenty of information about these diabolic cancer cells. How do they behave, how do they think, how do they act, what strengthens them and what makes them weak. Body dehydration seems to provide the perfect environment for the development of cancer cells. They are not friendly to oxygen and they love acidic environments. Oxygen who enters with water proved to be one of the best armor against cancer for prevention and cure. In fact I clearly remember that my mother was not drinking any water most of the day when she was younger and most of the time she was forcing herself to. What a puzzle! All the pieces where going one after the other into their place.

I came across this unique life story of Dr. Batmanghelidj in 1979 when he was put in Evin Prison for political reasons. There, he had a lot of fellow prisoners patients but not any medicine source but only water. He treated 3,000 prisoners mainly suffering from stress – induced peptic ulcer disease and under this uneasy circumstances a huge research based on water had started. It is remarkable and worth mentioning that although he was released from prison, he asked to stay there for an extra four-month period in order to cure more people. Specifically the combination of plenty of water with Himalayan pink salt, the purest salt on earth, is recommended as one of the best natural medicines against cancer and as a pain reliever in general. Himalayan salt used to be exchanged with gold in the days of Alexander the great. It is found in the ground and it is not passing under any other processing, it contains all natural elements identical to the elements contained in our body and it provides multiple benefits for our health.

CHAPTER THREE

Some say that universe is sending us clear signs and directions about our wonderings. What we have to do is only to ask. A few days after my mothers operation and while she was still in hospital I met one of my friends. She is a Greek – American lady. She is one of these sleepless, very energetic people who changed her study specialization a couple of times in order to deal with something she would really love in life. There she is today, an astrologer and a successful businesswoman as well in the tourism industry, mother of two wonderful sweet children. Her name in Natalie and she is an extremely social person.

Although I was feeling calm, it seems that sadness was engraved on my face and I happen to be dressed in black which I was constantly avoiding, based on my spiritual beliefs about the impact of the colors on our aura. Natalie looked at me and said: Oh you look sad, you are so sad. Then she told me about two young people she knew, they were around thirty years old and they were diagnosed with cancer. Although they looked and felt healthy they passed away almost one year after they were announced their disease. She was right. That moment I realized how valuable the maintenance of an optimistic psychology for diseased people is, and how strong and defining the power of belief can be.

We all started treating my mother as if she was healthy. I allowed her to do some work at home and very often we used to take some really long walks which could last for hours from the house to the Parthenon area and even up to the Lycabetus hill. Also, I made sure that her mind was all time occupied with hundreds of things. At that time we also did the shopping of our lives. I think that at this time mother replaced entirely her wardrobe. Regarding cancer, we all were mentioning it as it was something that belonged to the past, a bad adventure that passed and gave us a good lesson for the future. During all this period I considered the greatest luck the fact that mother was among these people who really wanted to try and fight for life. In our lifetime, sometimes it happens to meet people who don't really try for themselves; they just count on other people, strong people and suck some of their strength and energy. When they are depressed, you can encourage them and make them feel much better. But it always lasts temporarily. After a few hours or one day these people that I use to call "energy suckers" come back and it seems that you never worked with them. They keep on complaining about their unfortunate life, about how unfair their family, their partners and their employers have been to them. It is obvious that no matter how hard you have tried to help them see things in an optimistic way, they insist on seeing a black background behind their lives and its like they are struggling for other peoples mercy, they feed themselves with rivers of that mercy. Thank God! Mother was from the other humankind. She always had that strong character, very determinative and facing everything as it was coming. Of course she also used to complain about things but most of her topics were so funny that I am planning to use them in the future as a laugh resource for a family comedy.

It is meaningless to believe that our health can be harmed only by the heredity coming with our genes and from the things we eat. Psychological issues might damage health as well. The way we handle stress, sadness, anger, hatred, desperation and other negative emotions will have an important impact for our health. Controlling our food, be loyal in healthy diets of organic foods, sleep eight hours daily, get vitamins and drink a lot of water is not enough when living a stressful life within a stressful society.

If you can control your diet, you ought to control your negative emotions. Negative emotions are toxic. By controlling our emotions we don't mean to freeze our feelings **and keep ourselves out of this world. Be generous by leaving happiness overflow you when it comes to you, but be stoic and even controlling with pain, stress and other negative emotions when they knock your door.** Hundreds of studies have taken place and thousands of books have been written about the key to happiness. It takes hard work with yourself in order to transform your pessimistic self to a new optimistic, happy one. I was speechless when realized that the biggest part of negative emotions within a person is being caused by non-existing reasons. We think that our angry friend is angry with us but he or she might be angry for other reasons like making a mistake in the office or because their favorite team lost at the football game. Only one thing is certain: that we really do not know anything!

Manage your thoughts as you manage your diet. Reverse your trends of pessimistic thinking to trends of optimistic thinking. Master your mind because the mind is the builder. I will not indicate the study of complicated theories, oriental religions or the purchasing of special equipment but something much more simple. Every time that a negative thought shows up and starts polluting you like a virus polluting your computer with all further negative emotions, fears, anger or depression do what you would do for your computer. Install an anti virus program made from you and for you. This application is based on some basic principles like analyzing our thoughts, where did they come from, how important is the role of our past experiences to the generation of a thought, is this driven by our fears, our self esteem or even from what we use to listen for years during our childhood and teenage time or even later. From the time we are infants our family in order to protect us; use to fill us with fears. Don't do this or that, don't go there, this or that will happen to you if you do that. After the do and don'ts our family starts filling us with the musts. You must do this or that because this is the right thing to do. If you watch carefully the speed at which these restrictions and advice come out, then you will realize that most parents do not even think or process them before they speak. This material is there routed in their minds just like a program in a hard disk of a computer.

I was born and raised in Greece, this historic country. Poets and history writers use to say that due to its beauty, its history and culture, its geographic location surrounded by sea it has always been a temptation for someone to conquer. Just like a distinguished, proud woman resisting to a man, this country never surrendered to any invasion in history without fighting and therefore she paid a high price. Greek history is crowded with wars, revolutions, heroes and difficult eras of abjection for the people. Foreign attacks probably did not seem to be enough for the Greeks and every time they won to a war their Mediterranean spirit leaded them to bloody civil wars in order for a political party to accomplish to become government and rule the country.

Although both of my parents were born after the world war and they didn't really face any of this hard war eras, you could clearly identify on them some of the fears that their parents had planted in them. I was born later on when the country was flourishing in a secure democracy status. I will never forget how valuable food was perceived by my grandparents, even when there was an abundance of it. How they appreciated the fact that every day goods were available to people in the super markets and how blessed was that era that we their grandchildren came in this world. My parents even if they did not have such memories they use to reproduce such statement as if they had their own experiences and although during my childhood I never heard about a child in my country starving to death, I clearly remember my father forcing me to eat because I was a really bad eater and my parents happen to believe that I might die. Later on when my first nephew came in this world and happen to have taken after me regarding his feeding habits, the doctors ensured my sister that no children will starve to death and when he is really hungry he will ask for food. Nature had taken care of it.

I made all this above parenthesis in order to explain the way that some thoughts are loaded in our minds and how tyrannical they work within us. Most of these thoughts/ memories are there useless and outdated just like an outdated program in our computer hard disk. What we have to do is remove it to the recycle bin. Start knowing ourselves and distinguishing what we really want, what is bothering and what is not, is a good start. If we start this process we will realize that thousands of times in our everyday life we react on a specific way to some circumstances because that is what we supposed to do, that is what people do, and we never really wonder is this really bothering me, is that kind of reaction representing what I am. If we accomplish to know ourselves, control the trash thoughts/memories replaying in our minds like an old radio therefore release ourselves from heavy, unwanted, bitter emotions then we have done the key actions to regain happiness. In scientific terms happiness is not toxic. Happiness is a cure for the body and the soul.

Helping my mother review her aspect of life was an adventure. You can change everything to a person from the dressing to the residence city but when it comes to the mind! All this procedure, all this time was a great lesson for me as well. Other people and life situations make us discover things about ourselves that we didn't even suspect before. This is a changing process for everybody. Working with the mind is a never-ending process. You have to work every day just like an athlete exercising to keep in shape. We do the same mistakes every day, we correct them and there they are again. Working with our minds has to be like breathing: continuous, necessary and vital.

EPILOGUE

A few days before her last routine test my mother had a dream. She saw herself sitting in her armchair next to the fireplace. Suddenly an ugly looking, terrifying creature, a beast showed up from the other side of the house snarling while approaching her. She was so terrified to watch it coming closer and closer. Then at the end when it was close enough still snarling it collapsed in front of her feet and dropped dead.

Then my mother woke up from the nightmare, the nightmare of the beast, the cancer beast. It was dead. It had expired. Then she went back to sleep and had a peaceful sleep. A few days later, we got her test results. She was CANCER FREE.

APPENDIXES

1. C vitamin

Correspondence to: Dr. Mark Levine, Molecular and Clinical Nutrition Section, Bldg. 10, Rm 4D52–MSC 1372, National Institutes of Health, Bethesda MD 20892–1372; MarkL@mail.nih.gov

Early clinical studies showed that high-dose vitamin C, given by intravenous and oral routes, may improve symptoms and prolong life in patients with terminal cancer. Double-blind placebo-controlled studies of oral vitamin C therapy showed no benefit. Recent evidence shows that oral administration of the maximum tolerated dose of vitamin C (18 g/d) produces peak plasma concentrations of only 220 μmol/L, whereas intravenous administration of the same dose produces plasma concentrations about 25-fold higher. Larger doses (50–100 g) given intravenously may result in plasma concentrations of about 14 000 μmol/L. At concentrations above 1000 μmol/L, vitamin C is toxic to some cancer cells but not to normal cells in vitro. We found 3 well-documented cases of advanced cancers, confirmed by histopathologic review, where patients had unexpectedly long survival times after receiving high-dose intravenous vitamin C therapy. We examined clinical details of each case in accordance with National Cancer Institute (NCI) Best Case Series guidelines. Tumour pathology was verified by pathologists at the NCI who were unaware of diagnosis or treatment. In light of recent clinical pharmacokinetic findings and in vitro evidence of anti-tumour mechanisms, these case reports indicate that the role of high-dose intravenous vitamin C therapy in cancer treatment should be reassessed.

Vitamin C: Cancer Cure? by Marie McCullough, Philadelphia Inquirer, 06.19.2006

Is mainstream medical science ignoring an inexpensive, painless, readily available cure for cancer?

Mark Levine mulls this loaded question.

The government nutrition researcher has published new evidence that suggests vitamin C can work like chemotherapy - only better. But so far, he hasn't been able to interest cancer experts in conducting the kind of conclusive studies that, one way or the other, would advance treatment.

"If vitamin C is useful in cancer treatment, that's wonderful. If it's not, or if it's harmful, that's fine, too," said Levine, a Harvard-educated physician at the National Institute of Diabetes and Digestive and Kidney Diseases. "The goal is: Find what's true. Either way, the public wins, clinicians win, and patients win."

If Linus Pauling, the two-time Nobel laureate turned vitamin C zealot, had taken an equally dispassionate stance 30 years ago, who knows where the vitamin would be in oncology today. Surely not where it is: a dubious alternative on the fringes of medicine, despite its continuing links to remissions and cures.

This is not about popping supplements. It's about putting high-dose vitamin C, or ascorbic acid, into a vein, which requires needles and trained professionals.

The distinction between oral and intravenous is crucial. The body automatically gets rid of extra C through urine. Levine's lab has shown that, at high concentrations, the vitamin is toxic to many types of cancer cells in lab dishes. But to get that much C into the body before it's eliminated, it must be put directly into the blood.

This may explain the defining setback of Pauling's crusade. He and his collaborator, Scottish surgeon Ewan Cameron, gave C intravenously and orally, and claimed many of their cancer patients lived surprisingly long and well. In the 1970s, two rigorous government studies intended to test their claims gave only pills - and found no benefits.

How could so many smart people, including Pauling, ignore a variable as basic as the body's ability to absorb and clear a drug?

"I don't want to impugn anyone," Levine said. "It's one of these things where somebody didn't ask the right questions."

So Levine keeps on, driven by the still-open question:

Can intravenous C do what even the costliest, most targeted, most effective therapies cannot: kill cancer cells without harming healthy ones?

500 oranges

Loretta Hill, 42, of Pittsgrove, Salem County, sits at a faux granite table, facing a TV, chatting with two other cancer patients in the Marlton office suite of family physician Vivienne Matalon.

Each patient is tethered to an intravenous bag of C and other nutrients hung above the table that will take 40 minutes to drip into them. The fee, not usually covered by insurance, is $110.

Hill can't prove that C saved her from colon cancer, but she fervently believes it has.

She was diagnosed in 2001, at age 38, after a sudden bout of rectal bleeding. She had surgery, radiation, two courses of chemo. Six months later, the cancer was back - but had spread to both lungs.

After those tumors were cut out, her oncologist offered irinotecan, which costs about $9,500 a week. But, she says, he held out little hope. He declined to be interviewed.

By then, Hill could barely function, much to the anguish of her husband and 9-year-old daughter.

When she heard about Matalon's ascorbate infusions, she figured, "If this doesn't work, at least I'll be in a better position for more chemo."

Today, almost four years later, Hill is in college part time, plays soccer, and has no signs of cancer. Her weekly C dosage has been cut to 30 grams - about 500 oranges' worth - but she has no plans to quit because her only side effects are "fabulous hair and skin."

Bill Nath, 69, a Wichita, Kan., businessman, is an even more provocative case.

In 1996, blood in his urine led to a diagnosis of bladder cancer. Tumors were invading the organ and surrounding muscle.

Nath consulted experts at four major cancer centers from Wichita to New York. All recommended chemo, radiation, and removal of all or part of the bladder. Total removal would include the prostate, adding risks of incontinence and impotence.

One specialist "said if I didn't remove the whole bladder, I would die," said Nath. "It was pretty traumatic."

Nath ultimately made a choice that seemed suicidal to his wife, friends, and doctors: to keep part of his bladder and forgo chemo and radiation.

Instead, he got 30 grams of C twice a week for three months, then every month or two for four years at the Center for the Improvement of Human Functioning in Wichita. It was founded by Hugh Riordan, a physician and friend of Pauling's, now deceased.

Today, a decade after his diagnosis, Nath is cancer-free.

Levine, in collaboration with National Cancer Institute pathologists, reexamined, then published Nath's case and two others from Riordan's center. While such "case reports" prove nothing, Levine hoped they would stir interest in reexamining ascorbate in oncology.

But as Nath has discovered, when it comes to C, people who hear hoofbeats look for zebras.

"Everybody thought I was crazy," he said. "Now they probably think... it's a miracle or something."

Not a miracle

Vitamin C is not miraculous, proponents say. Just as some people die despite standard treatment, some die despite ascorbate drips.

"We may not be able to affect the ultimate outcome," said Matalon, who sees about 15 ascorbate patients a week. "But I think we see a dramatic improvement in quality of life."

The problem is, anecdotes and impressions don't count. Skeptics ask: Where's the data on dosing and regimens, on tumor responses, on survival?

"As far as I know, that kind of registry just doesn't exist now, and it's a huge weakness of the movement," acknowledged Ron Hunninghake, chief medical officer at Riordan's center, which is starting a database.

In any case, as consumers clamor for alternative therapies, intravenous C is gaining fans. Reports of side effects are rare, and risky patients - with kidney problems or blood disorders - are easily screened out.

"Interest is definitely growing," said Kenneth Bock, physician and president of the American College for Advancement in Medicine, an alternative-medicine society that teaches ascorbate infusion protocols.

Interest is not growing, however, among mainstream oncologists, judging from conferences, publications, and interviews with some of them.

The National Cancer Institute, with a $5 billion budget, is not sponsoring studies of intravenous C. Neither is the National Center for Complementary and Alternative Medicine - although it is paying for cancer studies of the noni extract herbal supplement and Reiki energy healing. The American Cancer Society and the American Association of Clinical Oncologists warn patients against high-dose C, as do leading cancer centers such as the University of Pennsylvania's and Memorial Sloan-Kettering in New York.

Jeffrey White, director of the National Cancer Institute's office of cancer complementary and alternative medicine, said that he's tried to "generate awareness" of Levine's research, and believes it justifies more studies in humans. But White acknowledged that the NCI has rejected "a few" proposals for such studies.

At the prestigious Mayo Clinic in Rochester, Minn., oncologist Edward Creagan said the idea that intravenous, but not oral, levels are toxic to cancer is "an intriguing concept."

"However, my own belief is that the vitamin C story is really ancient history," he said. "It would be very difficult for patients and clinicians to mount a lot of enthusiasm for another vitamin C study."

It was Creagan and his Mayo colleague, Charles Moertel, since deceased, who in the 1970s conducted the two NCI-funded "clinical trials" that showed vitamin C pills were no better than placebo pills for cancer patients.

A clinical trial is considered ultra-reliable because it is designed to keep beliefs and hopes from slanting findings.

Pauling lobbied for a trial, then later contended that the Mayo researchers enrolled unsuitable patients. A second trial in response to Pauling's criticism also bombed. Again he faulted the Mayo oncologists. He also threatened a libel suit against a Rochester newspaper for the headline "Pauling Wrong on Vitamin C for Cancer," and accused the New England Journal of Medicine and the NCI of accepting a "fraudulent" study, according to Australian medical historian Evelleen Richards.

By then, Pauling advocated treating everything from the common cold to mental illness with vitamins and other substances he dubbed "orthomolecular," meaning "right molecule." To many colleagues, this genius and visionary, winner of the 1954 Nobel in chemistry and the 1962 Nobel Peace Prize for his antiwar work, had become a kook - "The Old Man and the C".

Decades later, both skeptics and fans of C are gun-shy about more trials.

"There's tremendous resistance to even test this," Levine said. "It's very hard to revisit something like this without data. Information is diamonds."

As the chief of the molecular and clinical nutrition section at the National Institute of Diabetes and Digestive and Kidney Diseases - hardly a hotbed of federal cancer research - Levine discovered some diamonds "by accident."

In the early 1990s, his lab began looking at how the concentration of a nutrient affects its function, and how the body gets the proper concentration.

"As part of those studies, we looked at how vitamin C is absorbed in the intestine," Levine said.

By 2000, when that work led to an increase in the U.S. recommended daily allowance of vitamin C, Levine had become an expert on ascorbate's "pharmacokinetics" - what the body does to the drug.

Consumers and scientists already knew that ascorbate was an "antioxidant," meaning it protects cells from reactive oxygen molecules - the same marauders that turn peeled apples brown and wet metal rusty.

Indeed, the reason the American Cancer Society and others discourage ascorbate megadoses is that a few studies of cells in dishes suggest C might protect cancer from oxidant damage. Chemotherapy and radiation work partly by intentionally unleashing this damage.

But Levine's lab-dish studies showed that ascorbate transforms from an antioxidant into just the opposite - an oxidant promoter - when it reaches high concentrations. At these levels, which are achievable in the body only intravenously, C acts like a toxic drug by generating hydrogen peroxide, a powerful oxidant used as a bleaching agent, an antiseptic, and even a World War II rocket fuel.

Still, the biochemistry was puzzling. Putting pure peroxide in the bloodstream can be fatal, so why did patients feel fine when the vitamin that produces it was dripped into their veins?

Levine's experiments offered possible answers. Vitamin C did not generate peroxide in blood, only in liquid such as that found in body cavities. Thus, in the body, intravenous C must seep out of the blood to work.

Five out of nine types of cancer cells that were put in simulated body-cavity fluid died when concentrated ascorbate or peroxide was added to the dish. And the best part: This same lethal marinade had no effect on healthy cells.

For some reason, cancer cells were like the Wicked Witch of the West splashed with water - powerful villains vanquished by a mundane substance that is harmless to good guys.

Previously, Riordan had speculated that this was partly because an enzyme that neutralizes peroxide is abundant inside normal cells, and scarce inside cancerous ones. But by inducing cells to take in C, Levine proved that the internal concentration doesn't matter; malignant cells withered only when C surrounded them.

Armed with this new evidence, a coterie of researchers - all associated with Pauling or his disciples - have recently obtained private funding for small trials of intravenous C.

University of Kansas Medical Center physician Jeanne Drisko has $375,000 for a trial of 30 ovarian cancer patients. In Montreal, McGill University oncologist Wilson Miller has $300,000 to find the maximum safe doses for treating various cancers.

Meanwhile, Levine is forging ahead with animal studies, trying to decipher the molecular magic of C's selective toxicity.

Does that mean he believes C is an unsung cancer weapon?

"I think that question is akin to 'Do you still beat your wife?' " he said. "The question I would ask is: Shouldn't we investigate the potential of ascorbate as a drug?... Let's not guess anymore. Let's be motivated by the truth."

JAOA • Vol 107 • No 6 • June 2007 • 212-213

LETTER

Phase 1 Trial of High-Dose Intravenous Vitamin C Treatment for Patients With Cancer

Christopher M. Stephenson, DO; Robert D. Levin, MD; Christopher G. Lis, MPH

Cancer Treatment Centers of America Midwestern Regional Medical Center Zion, Illinois

To the Editor: For more than 30 years, the medical profession has had lingering questions about the efficacy of vitamin C in cancer therapy. Initial clinical reports1 and early preclinical studies[2] indicated that vitamin C administered intravenously may have potential anticancer benefits. Yet, few definitive clinical reports supporting this finding have been published. Thus, in October 2006, Cancer Treatment Centers of America (CTCA) initiated a US Food and Drug Administration–approved phase 1 study of intravenous vitamin C for patients with solid tumors who have exhausted all other available treatments. The investigators include an osteopathic internist (C.M.S.), a medical oncologist (R.D.L.), and a clinical epidemiologist (C.G.L.).

High doses (30 g/m^2 to 130 g/m^2) of vitamin C are used to achieve blood levels greater than the 20 mM that have been reported to be cytotoxic to tumor cells grown in hollow fibers.[3] Neil H. Riordan, PA-C, and colleagues,[4] reported that vitamin C infusions of 60 g resulted in brief blood level elevations to 24 mM. Blood levels are only elevated 0.2 mM when vitamin C is given orally. In the CTCA study, the first cohort of 3 patients is being treated with 30 g/m^2 — approximately 50 g for an average-sized individual — vitamin C infusions on 4 consecutive days per week for a period of 4 weeks.

Doses of vitamin C will be increased incrementally in future cohorts until the maximum tolerated dose is reached. Our goal is to have six dose escalations involving 18 patients. We are attempting to determine the safety, tolerability, optimum therapeutic dose, and pharmacokinetic profile of intravenous vitamin C, in addition to evaluating patient quality of life during treatment. We will also assess patients' tumor burden for preliminary indications of intravenous vitamin C anticancer activity. Information from this study may provide the basis for a phase 2 trial of intravenous vitamin C.

The phase 1 clinical trial is open for accrual. As of February, 3 patients in the first cohort had completed their 4-week series of vitamin C infusions. One of these patients, whose disease was in stable condition, wanted to continue the vitamin C infusions and is currently on a continuation protocol. We are actively recruiting the second cohort of 6 patients. The current study should resolve some critical unanswered questions about the efficacy of vitamin C in cancer care.

http://clinicaltrials.gov/ct2/show/NCT00441207

Study of High-Dose Intravenous (IV) Vitamin C Treatment in Patients With Solid Tumors

This study is currently recruiting participants.

Verified by Cancer Treatment Centers of America, August 2007

Sponsored by:	Cancer Treatment Centers of America
Information provided by:	Cancer Treatment Centers of America
ClinicalTrials.gov Identifier:	NCT00441207

Purpose

The primary purpose of this study is to evaluate the safety and tolerability of vitamin C (ascorbic acid) given by injection into the vein.

The second and third purpose of conducting this study is to observe
any evidence of tumor response to the vitamin C and compare the
level of fatigue (weakness), pain control, ability to do things, and
quality of life, before and after vitamin C is given.

Condition	Intervention	Phase
Cancer	Drug: Ascorbic Acid	Phase I

MedlinePlus related topics: Cancer

Drug Information available for: Ascorbic acid

U.S. FDA Resources

Study Type:	Interventional
Study Design:	Treatment, Non-Randomized, Open Label, Uncontrolled, Single Group Assignment, Safety/Efficacy Study
Official Title:	A Phase I Study of High-Dose IV Vitamin C Treatment in Patients With Solid Tumors

Further study details as provided by Cancer Treatment Centers of
America:

Primary Outcome Measures:

Evaluate the safety and tolerability of high dose IV vitamin C as a
monotherapy

Evaluate the pharmacokinetic profile of IV vitamin C at varying doses

Secondary Outcome Measures:

Determine if vitamin C accumulates with repeated daily therapy by measuring peak and nadir levels

Evaluate patient quality of life

Observe patients for clinical and radiological evidence of anti-tumor activity at the end of treatment

Estimated Enrollment:	18
Study Start Date:	August 2006
Estimated Study Completion Date:	August 2009

Detailed Description:

Preclinical studies of pharmacologic doses of vitamin C (ascorbic acid, ascorbate) have shown significant anticancer effects in animal models and tissue culture investigations including cytotoxic effects in certain cancer cell lines at micromolar to millimolar concentrations.

Early clinical studies have shown that intravenous and oral doses of vitamin C may improve symptoms and prolong survival in terminal cancer patients. More recent double-blind placebo-controlled studies have shown that oral adminstration of vitamin C provides no benefit to cancer patients. Conversely, intravenous vitamin C administration raises plasma concentrations as high as 14 mM/L, and concentrations of 1-5 mM/L have been found to be selectively cytoxic to tumor cells in vitro.

The proposed Phase I trial with vitamin C should achieve millimolar concentrations of vitamin C that have been shown to kill tumor cells in vitro. The maximum tolerated dose (MTD), PK, possible drug accumulation with repeated dosing, quality of life, pain response, fatigue status, and hints of efficacy in patients with advanced cancer will be examined.

Eligibility

Ages Eligible for Study:	18 Years and older
Genders Eligible for Study:	Both
Accepts Healthy Volunteers:	No

Criteria

Inclusion Criteria:

Primary histological diagnosis of advanced solid tumors (stage 3 and 4) and measurable disease.

Disease must have progressed for which no available treatment provides clinical benefit.

18 years of age or older.

No scheduled cancer therapy (chemotherapy, hormonal therapy, immune therapy, or radiation therapy) for three months after study entry, and the subject must have had their last therapy at least four (4) weeks prior to entry to this study.

Eastern Cooperative Oncology Group (ECOG) performance status of 0 to 2.

Informed Consent - The patient must be willing and able to sign the informed consent prior to the start of the trial.

Willingness to comply with the weekly phone calls between office visits.

Willingness to undergo central line placement (e.g., port-a-catheter, central venous catheter, percutaneously inserted central catheter [PICC] line placement) and able to manage care of the entry site safely.

Patients must be able to take food orally or have peg tube for feeding.

Life expectancy of at least 3 months.

Exclusion Criteria:

Glucose-6-phosphate dehydrogenase deficiency (G6PD) (a relative contraindication)

Renal insufficiency as evidenced by serum creatinine of 1.3 mg/dl or evidence of oxalosis by urinalysis.

Chronic hemodialysis.

Iron overload (a ferritin > 500 ng/ml).

Wilson's disease.

Compromised liver function with evidence of complete biliary obstruction or have a serum bilirubin of 2.0 or liver function tests (AST > 63, ALT > 95) exceeding 1.5 x the upper limit of normal.

Pregnant or lactating female.

Current tobacco use.

Evidence of significant psychiatric disorder by history or examination that would prevent completion of the study or preclude informed consent.

Aspirin use exceeding 325 mg per day.

Acetaminophen use exceeding 2 g per day.

Brain metastases that have not responded to therapy.

Contacts and Locations

Please refer to this study by its ClinicalTrials.gov identifier: NCT00441207

Contacts

Contact: Kathleen Katrenick	847-342-7475	kathleen.katrenick@ctca-hope.com
Contact: Candi Pfeiffer, RN	847-872-4015	candi.pfeiffer@ctca-hope.com

Locations

United States, Illinois
CTCA @ Midwestern Regional Medical Center   Recruiting
Zion, Illinois, United States, 60099
Principal Investigator: Christopher M Stephenson, DO
Principal Investigator: Robert D. Levin, MD
Principal Investigator: Christopher G. Lis, MPH

Sponsors and Collaborators

Cancer Treatment Centers of America

More Information

No publications provided

Study ID Numbers:	CTCA 06-04, Ascorbic Acid Injection
Study First Received:	February 26, 2007
Last Updated:	August 24, 2007
ClinicalTrials.gov Identifier:	NCT00441207 history of changes since first registered
Health Authority:	United States: Food and Drug Administration

Keywords provided by Cancer Treatment Centers of America:

IV	Ascorbic	Acid
IV	Vitamin	C
Cancer		
Advanced Solid Tumors		

Study placed in the following topic categories:

Antioxidants
Vitamins
Trace   Elements
Micronutrients
Ascorbic Acid

Additional relevant MeSH terms:

Molecular Mechanisms of Pharmacological Action
Growth Substances
Physiological Effects of Drugs
Protective Agents
Pharmacologic Actions

ClinicalTrials.gov processed this record on February 24, 2009

2. Vitamin B17 – Apricot Seeds

http://www.apricotseeds.com.au/Metabolic%20Therapy.pdf
40 pages for apricot seeds from G.Edward Griffin

http://www.worldwithoutcancer.org.uk./
http://www.whale.to/m/binzel.html
the book by Binzel called alive and well
Laetrile and the Life Saving Substance Called Cyanide
by Philip Binzel, Jr., M.D.
A doctor from the U.S. FDA once said that Laetrile contains "free"
   hydrogen cyanide and, thus, is toxic. I would like to correct that mis-
   conception:

There is no "free" hydrogen cyanide in Laetrile. When Laetrile comes
in contact with the enzyme beta-glucosidase, the Laetrile is broken
down to form two molecules of glucose, one molecule of benzaldehyde and one molecule of hydrogen cyanide (HCN). Within the
body, the cancer cell-and only the cancer cell-contains that enzyme.
The key word here is that the HCN must be FORMED. It is not
floating around freely in the Laetrile and then released. It must be
manufactured. The enzyme beta glucosidase, and only that enzyme,
is capable of manufacturing the HCN from Laetrile. If there are no
cancer cells in the body, there is no beta-glucosidase. If there is no
beta-glucosidase, no HCN will be formed from the Laetrile (1).

Laetrile does contain the cyanide radical (CN). This same cyanide radical is contained in Vitamin B12, and in berries such as blackberries,
blueberries and strawberries. You never hear of anyone getting
cyanide poisoning from 12 or any of the above-mentioned berries,
because they do not. The cyanide radical (CW) and hydrogen
cyanide (HCN) are two completely different compounds, just as
pure sodium (Na+) - one of the most toxic substances known to
mankind - and sodium chloride (NaCl), which is table salt, are two
completely different compounds.

If the above is true, how did the story ever get started that Laetrile contains "free" hydrogen cyanide? It was the Food and Drug Administration.

1. For a more detailed analysis of the theoretical action of Laetrile
against cancer cells, see G. Edward Griffin, World Without Cancer
(Thousand Oaks, CA: American Media, 1974).

I remember reading in some newspaper back in the late 1960's or early
1970's a news release from the FDA. This release stated that there
were some proponents of a substance known as "Laetrile" (I'd

never heard of it before) who were saying that this substance was capable of forming hydrogen cyanide in the presence of the cancer cell. The release continued by saying that, if this were actually true, we had, indeed, found a substance, which was target-specific, and would be of great value to the cancer patient. But, the news release went on to say, the FDA had done extensive testing of this substance, "Laetrile," and found no evidence that it contained hydrogen cyanide or that any hydrogen cyanide was released in the presence of the cancer cell. Thus, they said, Laetrile was of no value.

When it was clearly established some time later that Laetrile did, indeed, release hydrogen cyanide in the presence of the cancer cell, how do you suppose the FDA reacted? Did they admit that they were wrong? Did they admit that they had done a very inadequate job in running their tests? No! They now proclaimed that Laetrile contained hydrogen cyanide and thus was toxic!

So, here is a bureau of the Federal Government which, a short time before, had said that the reason Laetrile did not work was because it did not release hydrogen cyanide in the presence of cancer cells. Now, when they find that it does, they say that it is toxic. When offered an opportunity to present evidence of Laetrile's toxicity in Federal Court, they admitted that they had none.

NATURAL SOURCE

Laetrile is not a miracle drug. It is simply a concentrated form of Nitriloside. Amygdalin (Laetrile / Vitamin B17) is particularly prevalent in the seeds of those fruits in the Prunus Rosacea family (bitter almond, apricot, blackthorn, cherry, nectarine, peach and plum.) It is found in natural foods which contain nitriloside and

has been used and studied extensively for well over 100 years. It is
also contained in grasses, maize, sorghum, millet, cassava, linseed,
apple seeds, and many other foods that, generally, have been
deleted from the menus of modern civilization. Fruit kernels or
seeds generally have other nutrients as well, some protein, unsaturated fatty protein, unsaturated fatty acids, and various minerals. The most common source of B17 is the apricot kernel and is
present in about a 2-3 percent levels of concentration within the
seed kernel.

So there is no confusion please note; there are 3 names which are in-
terchangeable being Vitamin B17, Laetrile and Amygdalin. Vitamin B17 was the name given to the purified form of Amygdalin by
a Bio Chemist named Ernst T Krebs in 1952. He also called it
Laetrile which is simply short for Lavo-mandelonitrile and was
awarded its vitamin status officially in 1952 after advice from Dr
Dean Burke who was the co-founder of the National Cancer Institute. Amygdalin on the other hand is said to have been first discovered and used by a German chemist Leibig as far back as 1830. So,
laetrile/Vitamin B17 on the other hand is simply a more soluable
and concentrated form of amygdalin which allows it to be administered in a much greater concentration. Either way all 3 are essen-
tially the same thing.

Vitamin B17 / Laetrile is probably one of the most controversial medical topics in the last 30 years. You may remember back in the 50's
- mid 70's there was a lot hype in the medical world regarding a new
natural cancer treatment that was discovered that killed cancer cells.
This was the result of Dr Ernst Krebs findings and his research in a
book called World Without Cancer. Well after several years of court

cases and controversy regarding Laetrile it was finally stamped out by the FDA and reported to the mass media in the US as a fraud and failure. They called it Quackery in those days.

TODAY the hype has and is starting again as a result of **THE IN-TERNET**. The internet has allowed us to gain information from all over the world on what perhaps really happened.

So how does B17 kill cancer?...... Here we go....

Firstly we need to understand that our bodies use several enzymes to perform many tasks. Our body has one particular enzyme called Rhodanese which is found in large quantities throughout the body but is not present where ever there are cancer cells. Yet, where ever you find cancer in the body, you find another enzyme called Beta-Glucosidase. So, we have the enzyme Rhodanese found everywhere in the body except at the cancer cells, and we have the enzyme Beta-Glucosidase found in very large quantities only at the cancer cell but not found anywhere else in the body. If there is no cancer in the body there is no enzyme Beta-Glucosidase.

Now the following is what scares most people. You see, Vitamin B17 is made up of 2 parts glucose, 1 part Hydrogen Cyanide and 1 part Benzaldehyde (analgesic/painkiller). So its very important you understand the following:

When B17 is introduced to the body, it is broken down by the enzyme Rhodanese. The Rhodanese breaks the Hydrogen Cyanide and Benzaldehyde down into 2 by-products, Thiocyanate and Benzoic acid which are beneficial in nourishing healthy cells and forms the metabolic pool production for vitamin B12. Any excess of these by-products is expelled in normal fashion from the body via urine. Vitamin B17 passes through your body and does not last longer than 80 minutes inside your body as a result of the Rhodanese breaking it down. (Hydrogen Cyanide has been proven to be chemically inert and non toxic when taken as food or refined pharmaceutical such as laetrile. Sugar has be shown to be 20 times more toxic than B17.

HERE IS THE GOOD PART - When the B17 comes into contact with cancer cells, there is no Rhodanese to break it down and neutrelise it but instead, only the enzyme Beta-Gucosidase is present in very large quantities. When B17 and Beta-Glucosidase come into contact with each other, a chemical reaction occurs and the Hydrogen Cyanide and Benzaldehyde combine synergistically to produce a poison which destroys and kills the cancer cells.

This whole process is known as selective toxicity. Only the cancer cells are specifically targeted and destroyed.

Good & Bad Cyanide?

We all know that cyanide is bad for you, yet here we are jumping up and down saying its good for you because it kills cancer. Lets look at the real story.

Hydrogen Cyanide must be FORMED!! There is no free Hydrogen Cyanide in laetrile floating around freely in our body waiting to harm us when we eat apricot seeds or take laetrile. The enzyme Beta-Glucosidase, and only that enzyme is capable of manufacturing and forming the Hydrogen Cyanide from Laetrile. If there are no cancer cells in the body, there is no beta-glucosidase. If there is no beta-glucosidase, no hydrogen cyanide will be formed from laetrile. Even if there were some other way to manufacture cyanide from laetrile in the body, the amount would be so minute it would have little, if any toxic effect.

Laetrile does on the other hand contain the cyanide radical (CN-). So does Vitamin B12, Cassava and strawberries and a host of other foods we consume. You never heard of anyone getting cyanide poison from vitamin B12 or from eating strawberries because it just does not happen. Lets also look at table salt which is made up of sodium Chloride (NaCl) and is very common in most households. Yet, did you know pure sodium (Na+) is one of the most toxic substances known to man? Yet in their form locked together they are not toxic. Any good toxicologist will tell you sugar is 20 times more toxic than laetrile and salt is also much more toxic.

Now, here is the irony of all of this. Milligram for milligram, the chemotherapeutic agents which are commonly used in the treatment of cancer today, are hundreds of times more toxic than laetrile.

The best way to prove or disprove the vitamin B17 theory of cancer, would be to take several thousands of people, over a period of many years, expose them to a consistent diet of B17 rich nitriloside foods and then check the results. Fortunately this has already occurred by the study of the following cultures; The Hunza, aboriginal Eskimos, Hopi and Navajo Indians, Abkhazians.

HUNZA

In the remote recesses of the Himalayan Mountains, between West Pakistan, India and China there is a tiny Kingdom called Hunza. These people are known world over for their amazing longevity and health. They live well beyond 100 years and have commonly been known to still father children at the age of 110. One of the first medical teams to study the Hunza was headed by world-renown British surgeon Dr Robert McCarrison. Writing in the AMA Journal Jan 7, 1922 he reported:

"The Hunza has no known incidence of cancer. They have an abundant crop of apricots. These they dry in the sun and use largely in their food".

It is interesting to note that the traditional Hunza Diet contains over 200 times more nitriloside (B17 Rich food) than the average American or Australian Diet. There is no such thing as money in Hunza. A mans wealth is measured by the number of apricot trees he owns. And the most prized of all foods was considered to be the apricot seed. It is very common for the Hunza to eat between 30 - 50 (ie. about 30mg of B17) apricot seeds as an after lunch snack. The thousands of seeds they do not eat they store or grind them very finely and then squeezed under pressure to produce a very rich oil used in cooking and to apply to the skin. The apricot is staple food in Hunza. They use the apricot, its seed and the oil for practically everything. In addition to the ever present apricot, the hunzahuts eat mainly grain and fresh vegetables. These include buckwheat, millet, alfalfa, peas, broad beans, turnips, lettuce, sprouting pulse and berries of various sorts. All of these with the exception of lettuce and turnips contain vitamin B17.

It is important to know when the Hunza leave their secluded land and adopt the menus of other countries, they soon succumb to the same diseases and infirmities including cancer as the rest of man kind.

ESKIMOS

The Eskimos are another people that have been observed by medical teams for many decades and found to be totally free of cancer. The traditional Eskimo diet is amazingly rich in B17 nitrilosides that come from the residue of of the meat of caribou and other grazing animals, and also from the salmon berry. Another Eskimo delicacy is green salad made out of the stomach contents of caribou and reindeer which are full of fresh tundra grass. Tundra grasses such as Arrow are have shown to be contain the highest content of B17 than other grasses.

Alaska's most famous doctor Dr Preston A Price claims that, "In his 36 years of contact with these people he had never seen a single case of malignant disease among the truly primitive Eskimos, although it frequently occurred when they were modernized.

An interesting point to note is that when an Eskimo leaves his traditional way of life and begins to rely on a western/modern diet he becomes even more cancer prone than the average American.

HOPI & NAVAJO INDIANS

The Indians of North America are another people who are remarkably free from cancer. The AMA went as far as conducting a special study in an effort to discover why there was little to no cancer amongst the Hopi and Navajo Indians. The February 5, 1949 issue of the journal of the American Medical Association declared that they found 36 cases cases of malignant cancer from a population of 30,000. In the same population of white persons there would have been about 1800. Dr Krebs research later found that the typical diet for the Navajo and Hopi Indian consisted of nitriloside-rich foods such as Cassava. He calculated that some of the tribes would ingest the equivalent of 8000mg of Vitamin B17 per day from their diet!!!

ABKHAZIANS

The Abkhazians are found deep in the Caucasus Mountains on the Northwest side of the Black Sea. They are a people with almost the exact same health record and longevity as the Hunzakuts. Their food and lifestyle having to live in a harsh rugged terrain are almost identical. They follow a diet which is low in carbohydrates, high in vegetable proteins and rich in minerals and vitamins, especially vitamin B17.

Seeds Hold The Germ Of Life

This article is about the goodness of seeds and why you should include them in your daily diet.

Modern diets ignore the axiom that seeds hold the germ of life. Too often overlooked is the fact that nature has placed in seed foods the concentrated essence of all nutrition in order to provide nourishment for the sprouting plant. Only one part of any plant is outstandingly rich in protein and that is the seed. Proteins are centered in the seeds of a plant, so that the new life may receive ample nourishment for normal growth. Science has isolated and identified most of the nutrients in seed foods. It is my belief that seed foods contain life-sustaining powers which are, as yet, unknown to science, and from which we can benefit greatly when these seeds are made a part of our daily diets. Little by little, modern nutritional science is inclining to the belief that whole seed cereals (I stress 'whole' because of the health-blind custom of milling most of the food value out of our cereals) can supply for your diet a now missing something that formerly was there when life and eating habits were much closer to the primitive. In fact, several biochemists have told me it's their private opinion that only when we regain that missing 'something' in our diets which the primitive peoples enjoyed will we find the preventive for many of our deficiency and wasting diseases. Seed foods have always formed a large portion of the instinctive diet followed by primitive peoples. And so highly did they value these seed foods that many religious superstitions grew up around them.

For instance, the Indians of the twoAmerican continents, from Alaska
to Patagonia, placed bowls of cereal grains and sunflower seeds on
the graves of their dead for food to nourish them on their long, dangerous journey into the next world. What had been good, energy-
giving food while they were alive, the surviving Indians reasoned,
must also be good food for them when dead. How many times this
past year has your table been graced with millet, steel-cut oats,
whole unbolted cornmeal, raw wheat germ, sesame seed or sunflower seed? Have your morning pancakes and your suppertime
muffins been made with all-starch white flour or devitalized corn
meal-or with whole wheat flour and millet meal? Does your cereal
bowl at breakfast contain a no-food-value, devitalized dry cereal-
or does it contain steel-cut oats, or millet meal mush? Were the
cookies you carried in your lunch topped with white sugar, or with
sesame seeds?

Never mind answering! Unless you are one of the disturbingly small
minority in this country who recognizes the stay-young values in
seed cereals, I know that your pancakes were made with 100 per
cent-starch white flour; that your muffins were made with devitalized corn meal; that your cereal bowl contained a patented dry cereal, one of the biggest frauds in modern nutrition; and that your
cookies were made with more white flour and decorated with no-nu-
trition white sugar. And yet you wonder why your hair turns gray
(when it doesn't fall out altogether), why your muscles grow flabby,
your figure becomes lumpy, your teeth decay, your eyesight grows
poorer all the time, your sexual powers disappear prematurely and
your nerves act like Mexican jumping beans. Much talk is in the air
these days about 'miracle foods.' Two of the so-called 'miracle
foods' most widely advertised are brewers' yeast and blackstrap mo-

lasses. Heaven alone knows how many hundreds of packages of these two unpalatable products are lying around on cupboard shelves, untouched after the first few attempts to get them down. No food can work 'miracles' for your health if you don't like it well enough to eat it regularly.

I don't deny that brewers' yeast and blackstrap molasses contain all the nutrients attributed to them. But why fool yourself that you're obtaining the benefits of the valuable nutrients in these two products, when actually you can't tolerate the stuff enough to eat it regularly, no matter how you may try to disguise it? How much better it would be for your stay-young efforts if you were to depend instead on the equally valuable nutrition to be found in seed cereals that not only nourish you with an abundance of the same proteins, minerals and vitamins, but which taste good besides. Let me introduce you to several of the new-old seed cereals about which you probably know very little. Of course, there's no need to go into details on such seed foods as nuts (don't overlook the splendid nutrition and taste enjoyment of fresh coconut as bought in the shell, or in packages at health food stores-not the desiccated, long-keeping, artificially sweetened variety found on grocery shelves) peas and beans. These foods are too well known to need any introduction. They all contain a fair quality of vegetable protein, besides essential minerals and vitamins. And if you find them easy to digest (many persons do not), then by all means include them in your daily diet.

The three seed cereals with which I wish to acquaint you are both satisfying and easily digestible. They merit a place in every diet, for gradually they will take away your desire for white breads and rich pastries. And after you've succeeded in eliminating all artificial, pure-starch, youth-destroying foods from your diet, your body will show its gratitude by losing that bloated, flabby look which puts the years on you along with the pounds. Seed cereals and whole grains help build a body that is firm and lithe-a young body.

Millet

Millet is the first of the seed cereals that should be on your table regularly. Little known in this country, except as poultry and animal feed, millet has been one of the principal grains of Eastern Europe, Africa, Siberia and China for centuries. Five hundred years before the beginning of the modern Christian era, the Greek philosopher Pythagoras praised the high nutritive value of millet, and advised his followers (all vegetarians) to adopt millet as the mainstay of their diets. Contrary to popular belief, millet and not rice is the basic food of most Chinese in their native country. Only the small-statured, less robust Southern Chinese subsist on rice. The tall, sturdy, vigorous Northern Chinese have used millet as their principal food for many centuries. We Americans will adopt a certain plant from other con' tinents, but for our livestock, not for our own bodies. Our depraved appetites tend to spurn the wholesome, health-giving, youth-protective natural foods in favor of the widely advertised artificial foods that make old men and women of us in our prime.

On a Saturday morning not long ago, while driving to the West Coast, I stopped in a small Iowa town located in the heart of a rich farming section, and parked in front of the local grocery store. The street was lined with farmers' trucks and autos while the families went about their weekly shopping.

Before long the family in the car next to mine returned, loaded down with their purchases-the father carrying a sack labeled 'Whole Millet, Chicken Feed, Mineral-and-Protein Rich, For Laying Stock';

the children alternately lapping on ice cream cones or munching on candy bars; and the mother carrying a box of canned goods topped by two loaves of baker's white bread (even sliced for her) and a cellophane package of dried noodles. What a travesty on good nutrition! The only real nourishment in all their purchases-the whole millet-was going to their chickens, while the devitalized white-flour bread and noodles were supposed to 'nourish' the hard-working farmer and farm wife and their growing children. Watching them as they drove away, I could have wept for the long-life days when a farmer took his own grain to the mill to be ground whole, then returned it to the barrel in the pantry; and the farm wife made her own bread and noodles from the whole grain flour.Millet is one of the oldest and most nutritious foods known to man. It is a completely balanced grain, non-acid forming and rich in high-grade protein, minerals, vitamins and lecithin (the same tasty substance found in egg yolk, and containing that valuable B-vitamin, choline for its powers to prevent fatty deposits on artery walls).

Laboratory investigations have revealed that no food is digested with as great ease as millet. It does not ferment in the stomach, causing digestive and intestinal distress, as do the foods and breakfast cereals made from white flour and other devitalized grains.Millet is non-fattening, since it does not produce the excessive fat that follows a diet containing the all-starch, low-mineral, no-vitamin, devitalized corn, wheat and rice. To our own detriment, we have come to rely too heavily on wheat, corn and rice as our national cereals, forgetting that there are equally as tasty, and far more nutritious, seed foods which we should adopt for the sake of our own, and the national, health. After the First World War, millions of Russian peasants in

White Russia faced starvation. In desperation, they ate the millet which had been put away for the chickens they no longer had. And what happened? Not only did these peasants survive the long period of famine, but they soon discovered they were enjoying better health than they had ever known while consuming their former varied diets. One of the peasants, who had suffered from stomach ulcers for fifteenyears, found that his ulcers disappeared in six months on his forced diet of nothing but millet.

News of this millet diet gradually reached the scientists in this country. Professors Osborn and Mendel at Yale, after extensive experiments, announced that millet contains a richer store of vitamins than any other cereal in common use in the United States; that millet is the only grain capable of supplying all the vitamins needed for human nutrition. Later studies also revealed that millet contains every one of the 10 essential amino acids, and that its protein is equal in value to animal protein. Dr. John Harvey Kellogg declared that millet is the only cereal capable of supporting human life when used as the sole item in the diet. Of course, no one wants to live exclusively on millet-unless forced to do so as were those desperate Russian peasants. But if worse came to worst, scientists are convinced that you could live on a diet of nothing but millet, and not only survive, but become even healthier and more vigorous than you ever were. It would be unfortunate, indeed, if you tried to live on wheat alone, even whole wheat, since this grain lacks certain of the 10 essential amino acids. But the completeness and high quality of the proteins in millet make it possible for your body to be well supplied with all the essential amino acids, even though little or no other protein foods are eaten.

This is a fact which I believe should be more widely utilized by dietitians and homemakers during times of meat scarcities and meat rationing. During our past era of meat rationing, in the days of World War II, home economists promoted, as meat substitutes, rice, macaroni, spaghetti and noodle dishes. Starch is never a safe substitute for protein. The only foods which should ever appear in the menu as an honest substitute for a meat dish are eggs, cheese, milk and high-protein seed cereals. By adding extra amounts of dry skim milk (a rich source of protein) to these truly protein meat substitutes, a meatless diet may be prevented from falling far below a safe daily minimum of 100 to 150 grams of protein. Now don't get the idea that I'm recommending that you do away with meat in your diet, and substitute millet. Meat is an unexcelled, hard-to-replace food. But what I do want to impress upon you is this: If the meat situation again becomes 'tight,' remember that you can stretch your budget through liberal use of millet, a safe vegetable protein. Moreover, millet is almost a necessity in a vegetarian diet, because it can provide a complete protein without the need of eating a lot of bulk, something not true of most other vegetable proteins. If there were enough meat in this country, at a fair price for everybody, then I'd say 'meat twice a day, at least.' But we might as well face the fact that meat is deliberately kept high-priced and scarce in this country to benefit the interests of a selfish few, rather than priced reasonably enough so plenty of meat would be available to every pocketbook, thereby appreciably raising the national health standards. The short-sightedness of some high officials in pandering to the interests of the cattle industry prevents our importing enough meat to place at least one red meat dish on every table in the nation twice a day, seven days a week-and at a price well within reach of the lowest income group. This may sound like Utopia to you. But I saw first-grade meat being sold at phenomenally low prices in Uruguay and Argentina, as it always has been-and surely what these two sister countries can do, we in the great United States of America could also do for our own populace.

But it won't be done-you and I know that. In fact, the meat situation will probably be a lot worse before it gets better. And I realize there are thousands of persons living on incomes that won't permit their purchasing meat every day in the week. For that reason, I believe that more recognition should be given to millet (sunflower seeds, too) as a nutritionally safe, low-cost, easily digestible meat substitute. In addition, millet is an unusually rich source of riboflavin -one of the B-vitamins. This seed cereal also provides rich amounts of thiamin (B-i), and vitamins A and E, together with good amounts of the other B-complex factors. What's more, millet contains a good balance of all the minerals needed by the human body for optimum health.

We are specialized in anti-aging health products. Learn 'The Six Secrets To A Long Young Life'. To receive your free report visit our AntiAgingHealthProducts.com website and sign up for your free copy.

By Luzia Braun

Metabolic therapy is a non-toxic cancer treatment based on the use of Vitamin B- 17, proteolytic pancreatic enzymes, immuno-stimulants, and vitamin and mineral supplements.

Apricot seeds should be ground up in everything you eat. Anywhere up to 70 seeds per day. The FDA recommend not to ingest more than

6 seeds per hour because toxic reactions may occur, such as gastric upset, headache, vomiting and loose bowels. Many people take 15 seeds per day. Can skip a day and then take 40 the next day, and so on and so on. Bone cancer survivors take 5 seeds per waking hour with pancreatic enzymes, etc... (I'm sure not e v e r y hour). In general, take one apricot kernel for each 5 pound of body weight, daily. Example: 180 lb = 36 apricot seeds daily. Dr. Krebs recommends 30 to 35 seeds per day as nutritional support for clinical cancer sufferers. To start, it is recommended that along with the purified forms of B-17, either intravenous or oral, cancer patients eat one apricot seed for every 10 lbs of body weight. If this dosage is tolerated well, it may be increased to 30 to 35 kernels per day

"Chemotherapy and radiation do not make the body well. They destroy, they do not heal. The hope of the doctor is that the cancer will be destroyed without destroying the entire patient. These therapies do kill cancer cells, but they kill a lot of good cells too including the cells of the immune system, the very system that one NEEDS to get well. If a cancer patient survives the treatment with enough immune system left intact, the patient may appear to get well at least temporarily, but he will have sustained major damage to his body and his immune system. How much better it is to nourish the immune system directly by the use of natural therapies to assist it in getting you well instead of destroying it by the use of these therapies. **Then the immune system itself can kill the cancer cells without any side effects and heal your body at the same time." Dr. Lorraine Day, M.D.** Dr. Day is an internationally acclaimed orthopedic trauma surgeon and best selling author was for 15 years on the faculty of the University of California, San Francisco School of Medicine as Associate Professor and Vice Chairman of the Department of Orthopedic Surgery. She was also Chief of Orthopedic Surgery at San Francisco General Hospital. In 1992, Dr. Day developed breast cancer, biopsy-proven, that become so severe it was eventually diagnosed as terminal. **But she refused chemotherapy, radiation and mutilating surgery because of their dangerous side effects and chose, instead, to get well by a totally natural Ten Step Health Plan. She continues to be totally well and cancer-free a full twelve years later.**

3. Water – Common Cause and Natural cure
http://www.naturalnews.com/Report_water_cure_0.html

http://www.watercure.com/
F. Batmanghelidg, M.D. Author of : Your body's Many Cries for Water, Obesity Cancer Depression, Their Common Cause & Natural Cure.

A FEW WORDS ABOUT THE AUTHOR

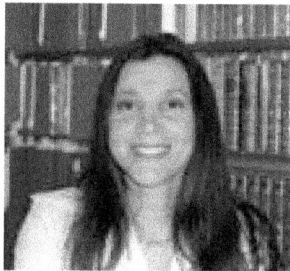

Maria D. Georga was born in the historic city of Sparta in Greece. She graduated from Greek and British universities and she holds BA & MBA degrees in Management, Business Administration, Human Resources Management with specialization in Employment Relations. For almost fourteen years she worked as an executive for various international companies. From 2007 she is an entrepreneur acting mainly in the Health tourism industry and in business consulting. She is a deeply spiritual person and she is involved with religions and spiritual theories.

"Killing the Cancer Beast" is the first of her books that she decided to publish. It is based on the real story of her mother's fight with cancer. Significant part of the sale of each book will be given to hospitals, organizations and scientists involved with research regarding cancer cure.